CHAIR YOGA BOOK FOR SENIORS OVER 60

How To Improve Balance, Mobility, Posture And Loss Weight While Reclaiming Independence

Samantha Lee Smith

COPYRIGHT

[Copyright 2024] by Anna Smith Tom

This publication is intended for informational purposes only. The information provided is not a substitute for professional medical advice, diagnosis, or treatment. Always seek the advice of your physician or other qualified health provider with any questions you may have regarding a medical condition. Never disregard professional medical advice or delay in seeking it because of something you have read in this publication.

DISCLAIMER

This chair yoga book for seniors over **60** is intended for informational purposes only and should not be considered a substitute for professional medical advice, diagnosis, or treatment. The exercises and information provided in this book are meant to be gentle and accessible for seniors, but it is important for individuals to consult with their healthcare provider before beginning any new exercise program, including chair yoga. The author and publisher are not liable for any injuries or damages that may occur as a result of practicing the exercises or following the advice in this book. Each individual's health and fitness level are unique, and it is essential to listen to your body and modify exercises as needed to ensure safety and comfort. By using this book, readers acknowledge and accept responsibility for their own health and well-being.

ABOUT THE AUTHOUR

I'm Samantha Lee Smith, and I'm thrilled to share my passion for chair yoga with seniors over 60. As a certified yoga instructor specializing in senior wellness, I've seen firsthand the transformative power of yoga in improving physical health and mental well-being. My journey into yoga began years ago when I discovered its profound benefits for my own body and mind. As a senior I knew I should be more intentional with my fitness journey. Since then, I've dedicated myself to helping others experience the joy and vitality that yoga can bring, regardless of age or ability.

My inspiration for writing this book stemmed from a desire to make yoga accessible to everyone, especially seniors who may face mobility challenges or health concerns. I understand the importance of gentle movement and mindfulness practices for maintaining overall health and quality of life as we age. Through my work with seniors in community centers, retirement homes, and private sessions, I've witnessed the profound impact that chair yoga can have on improving flexibility, reducing pain, and fostering a sense of connection and empowerment.

In this book, I've carefully curated a collection of chair yoga poses, breathing exercises, and relaxation techniques specifically tailored to the needs and abilities of seniors over 60. My goal is to provide clear, easy-to-follow instructions that anyone can use to start their own chair yoga practice, whether at home or in a group setting. I've also included safety tips, modifications, and encouragement to help readers feel confident and supported on their yoga journey.

As an advocate for holistic wellness, I believe that yoga is not just about physical exercise but also about cultivating inner peace, resilience, and joy. Through chair yoga, seniors can tap into their innate strength and vitality....

UNDERSTANDING CHAIR YOGA

Let's talk about chair yoga. It's something really cool that I've been learning about, and I want to share it with you because it's made such a big difference in my life and over 3000 seniors worldwide . Chair yoga is like regular yoga, but it's done sitting down or holding onto a chair for support. It's perfect for people like me who might not be able to stand for long periods or get down on the floor easily.

So, what's the deal with chair yoga? Well, it's all about taking care of our bodies and minds, especially as we get a little older. You see, as we age, our bodies might not move the same way they used to. We might have achy joints, stiffness, or balance issues. That's where chair yoga comes in. It's gentle and safe, but still super effective at keeping us flexible, strong, and relaxed.

One of the best things about chair yoga is that you can do it anywhere – at home, at work, or even when you're out and about. All you need is a sturdy chair and a little bit of space to move your arms and legs. And don't worry if you're not super flexible or coordinated – neither am I! Chair yoga is all about doing what feels good for your body, so there's no need to push yourself too hard.

Now, let's talk about why chair yoga is so awesome. First off, it helps with flexibility. You know how sometimes it's hard to bend down to tie your shoes or reach for something on a high shelf? Chair yoga can help with that. By gently stretching and moving our bodies, we can improve our range of motion and make everyday tasks a little easier.

But flexibility is just the beginning. Chair yoga also helps with strength. You might not think that sitting in a chair could make you stronger, but it totally can! By doing simple exercises like lifting your legs or pushing your arms against the chair, you can build up your muscles and improve your overall strength and stability.

And let's not forget about relaxation. Life can be stressful sometimes, right? Well, chair yoga can help with that too. By focusing on our breath and taking slow, deep breaths, we can calm our minds and relax our bodies. It's like hitting the reset button on a hectic day.

So, that's chair yoga in a nutshell. It's a gentle, effective way to take care of our bodies and minds as we get older. And the best part? It's fun! So why not give it a try? Grab a chair and join me for a little yoga session. Trust me, you won't regret it!

What is Chair Yoga?

Chair yoga— it's my favorite way to stay healthy and happy, especially as a senior over 60. Chair yoga is like regular yoga, but with a twist— we get to do all the awesome poses while sitting comfortably in a chair! How cool is that?

Now, you might be wondering, "What exactly is chair yoga?" Well, let me break it down for you. Chair yoga is a modified form of yoga that's perfect for folks like us who might not be able to do all those fancy poses on a yoga mat. Instead, we use a chair for support and do all our stretching, twisting, and breathing right from our seats.

So, what kind of poses do we do in chair yoga? Oh, we do all sorts of fun stuff! We start by sitting tall in our chairs, feet flat on the ground, and we take big, deep breaths to center ourselves. Then, we might do some gentle stretches, like reaching our arms up to the sky or twisting our bodies from side to side. And don't forget about those leg stretches— lifting our knees up towards our chest or kicking our legs out in front of us feels amazing!

But chair yoga isn't just about stretching our bodies— it's also about calming our minds and finding inner peace. That's where the breathing comes in! We practice deep, slow breaths, inhaling through our noses and exhaling through our mouths. It's like a mini vacation for our brains!

Now, you might be thinking, "Can I really do chair yoga if I've never done yoga before?" Absolutely! Chair yoga is for everyone, no matter your age or experience level. You don't need to be super flexible or have perfect balance— all you need is a chair and a willingness to give it a try!

Before we get into our chair yoga practice, though, there are a few things to keep in mind. First, always listen to your body. If something feels uncomfortable or painful, stop and take a break. Second, go at your own pace. There's no rush, so take your time and enjoy the movements. And finally, don't forget to smile! Chair yoga is supposed to be fun and relaxing, so let your inner joy shine through!

So, there you have it— chair yoga in a nutshell! It's a fun, gentle way to stretch our bodies, calm our minds, and connect with our breath. Plus, it's a great way to meet new friends and feel part of a community. Ready to give it a try? Grab a chair and let's get started on our chair yoga journey together!

Benefits of Chair Yoga for Seniors

Let me tell you about all the amazing benefits of chair yoga for seniors like us! It's seriously awesome, and I can't wait to share it with you.

1. Improves Flexibility: Chair yoga helps keep our bodies flexible and nimble, even as we get older. The gentle stretches and movements help loosen up tight muscles and joints, making it easier to move around and do everyday activities.

2. Enhances Balance and Stability: One of the coolest things about chair yoga is how it helps improve our balance and stability. By practicing different poses while seated, we can strengthen our core muscles and improve our posture, which helps prevent falls and accidents.

3. Reduces Stress and Anxiety: Chair yoga is like a mini vacation for our minds! When we focus on our breath and move our bodies mindfully, it helps calm our nervous system and reduce stress and anxiety. It's like hitting the reset button on our day!

4. Boosts Mood and Well-Being: Doing chair yoga makes me feel happy and content. It releases feel-good chemicals in our brains called endorphins, which can lift our mood and give us a sense of inner peace and happiness.

5. Increases Energy Levels: Chair yoga might seem relaxing, but it's also super energizing! The gentle movements and deep breathing help improve circulation and oxygen flow throughout our bodies, giving us a natural energy boost.

6. Supports Joint Health: As we age, our joints can start to feel stiff and achy. But chair yoga can help! The gentle movements and stretches help lubricate our joints and reduce stiffness, keeping them healthy and pain-free.

7. Improves Sleep Quality: If you're like me and struggle with sleep sometimes, chair yoga might be just what you need. The relaxation techniques and calming poses can help quiet the mind and prepare the body for a restful night's sleep.

8. Increases Mindfulness and Awareness: Chair yoga teaches us to be present in the moment and pay attention to what's happening in our bodies and minds. This mindfulness practice can help us feel more connected to ourselves and the world around us.

9. Encourages Social Connection: Chair yoga classes are a great way to meet new friends and feel part of a community. Sharing the experience of yoga with others can create a sense of belonging and support.

10. Promotes Self-Care and Self-Love: Taking time out of our day to practice chair yoga is a form of self-care and self-love. It's a way to show ourselves kindness and compassion, both physically and emotionally.

This is just a few of the many benefits of chair yoga for seniors like us. It's not only good for our bodies but also for our minds and spirits. Ready to roll out that yoga mat— er, chair— and give it a try? I promise you won't regret it!

GETTING STARTED WITH CHAIR YOGA

Let's talk about how to get started with chair yoga— it's an exciting journey, and I'm here to guide you every step of the way. So, what do you need to get started? Let's break it down together!

1. A Comfortable Chair: First things first, you'll need a sturdy and comfortable chair to practice chair yoga. Choose a chair with a flat seat and a firm backrest for added support. Make sure it's a chair you feel safe and comfortable sitting in for an extended period.

2. Open Space: Find a quiet and open space in your home where you can practice chair yoga without any distractions. Clear away any clutter or obstacles to create a safe and inviting environment for your practice. It doesn't have to be a large space— just enough room to move your arms and legs freely.

3. Comfy Clothing: Wear loose, comfortable clothing that allows you to move freely and doesn't restrict your range of motion. Opt for breathable fabrics that won't make you feel too hot or sweaty during your practice. Remember, comfort is key!

4. Mindful Mindset: Before you begin your chair yoga practice, take a moment to set an intention or focus for your session. Maybe you want to feel more relaxed, energized, or centered. Whatever it is, bring that intention into your practice and let it guide you.

5. Breath Awareness: Throughout your chair yoga practice, pay attention to your breath. Take slow, deep breaths in through your nose and out through your mouth, allowing your breath to guide your movements. Notice how your body feels with each inhale and exhale, and use your breath to anchor yourself in the present moment.

6. Safety First: Always prioritize safety during your chair yoga practice. Listen to your body and honor its limitations— never force yourself into a pose that doesn't feel right. If something feels uncomfortable or painful, back off and modify the pose as needed. Remember, it's okay to take breaks and rest whenever you need to.

7. Gentle Warm-Up: Start your chair yoga practice with a gentle warm-up to prepare your body for movement. Roll your shoulders, stretch your arms, and gently twist your torso from side to side. Focus on loosening up any areas of tension or stiffness before moving into deeper stretches or poses.

8. Follow Along: Whether you're following a chair yoga video, attending a class, or using a guidebook, remember to follow along at your own pace. Don't worry about doing everything perfectly— just do what feels right for you in the moment. Allow yourself to explore and enjoy the journey of chair yoga without judgment or pressure.

9. Have Fun: Most importantly, have fun with your chair yoga practice! Let go of any expectations or worries and simply enjoy moving your body and connecting with your breath. Chair yoga is all about feeling good and taking care of yourself, so relax, smile, and embrace the experience.

So, there you have it— everything you need to get started with chair yoga! With a comfortable chair, an open space, and a mindful mindset, you're ready to embark on this wonderful journey of self-discovery and well-being. Are you excited? I know I am! Let's dive in and explore the amazing world of chair yoga together.

Setting Up Your Space

1. Find a Quiet Spot: First things first, find a quiet spot in your home where you can practice without any distractions. It could be a corner of your living room, a spot in your bedroom, or even a cozy area on your balcony— anywhere that feels peaceful and inviting.

2. Clear the Area: Next, clear away any clutter or obstacles from your chosen space. You want to have plenty of room to move around without bumping into furniture or tripping over objects. It's important to create a safe and open space for your practice.

3. Choose the Right Chair: Now, let's talk about your chair. Choose a sturdy and stable chair with a flat seat and a firm backrest for added support. Make sure the chair is at a comfortable height for you to sit in without feeling too low or too high off the ground.

4. Grab Some Props (Optional): If you have any props like yoga blocks, straps, or bolsters, feel free to grab them! Props can help enhance your practice and provide

additional support or assistance during certain poses. However, don't worry if you don't have any props— chair yoga can be done with just a chair!

5. Create a Cozy Atmosphere: Add some cozy touches to your space to make it feel extra inviting. You could light a scented candle, play some soft music, or hang up a string of fairy lights— whatever helps you feel relaxed and at ease.

6. Consider Lighting: Pay attention to the lighting in your space. Natural light is always best, so if possible, practice near a window where you can enjoy some sunlight. If natural light isn't available, you can use lamps or overhead lights to create a warm and inviting atmosphere.

7. Set the Mood: Before you begin your practice, take a moment to set the mood. Close your eyes, take a few deep breaths, and visualize yourself feeling calm, centered, and ready to practice. Setting an intention for your practice can help you stay focused and present throughout.

8. Personalize Your Space: Finally, don't forget to personalize your space to make it your own. Add some personal touches like a favorite blanket, a photo of loved ones, or a small plant to brighten up your practice area and make it feel like home.

Choosing The Right Chair

1. Sturdy and Stable: First things first, you'll want a chair that's sturdy and stable. Look for a chair with a solid frame and legs that won't wobble or tip over easily. This will help you feel safe and supported during your practice.

2. Flat Seat: Check to make sure the chair has a flat seat without any cushions or indentations. A flat seat provides a stable surface for sitting and moving during your practice. It allows you to maintain proper alignment and balance without sinking or sliding around.

3. Firm Backrest: Next, consider the backrest of the chair. Look for a chair with a firm backrest that provides good support for your spine. A supportive backrest helps you sit up tall and maintain proper posture throughout your practice.

4. Comfortable Height: Pay attention to the height of the chair. You'll want a chair that allows your feet to rest flat on the ground with your knees bent at a comfortable angle. Avoid chairs that are too low or too high, as they can cause discomfort and strain on your joints.

5. Armrests (Optional): Some chairs come with armrests, while others don't. It's a matter of personal preference whether you choose a chair with or without armrests for your practice. If you opt for armrests, make sure they're at a comfortable height and don't restrict your movement.

6. Size and Proportions: Consider the size and proportions of the chair in relation to your body. You'll want a chair that fits you well and allows you to sit comfortably without feeling cramped or squeezed. If possible, test out different chairs to find the one that feels just right for you.

7. Portability: Think about whether you'll be practicing chair yoga at home or on the go. If you plan to take your chair to different locations, you'll want a lightweight and portable option that's easy to transport. Look for chairs that are foldable or stackable for added convenience.

8. Personal Preference: Finally, trust your instincts and choose a chair that feels right for you. Whether you prefer a sleek modern design or a cozy cushioned seat, go with the chair that speaks to your heart and makes you excited to practice yoga.

Choosing the perfect chair for your chair yoga practice! With a sturdy frame, flat seat, firm backrest, and comfortable height, you'll be all set to dive into your practice and experience the joy of chair yoga. I can't wait for you to find the chair that's just right for you!

Picking The Right Outfit

1. Comfort is Key: First things first, I always prioritize comfort when picking out my yoga outfit. I want to wear something that feels soft and cozy against my skin, so I can focus on my practice without any distractions.

2. Choose Breathable Fabrics: When it comes to fabrics, I prefer breathable materials like cotton or bamboo. These fabrics help keep me cool and dry, even when I start to work up a sweat during my practice. Plus, they feel so nice and lightweight against my skin!

3. Opt for Loose-Fitting Clothing: I like to wear loose-fitting clothing for chair yoga, as it gives me plenty of room to move and stretch without feeling restricted. Baggy tops and pants allow me to bend and twist comfortably without any tightness or discomfort.

4. Consider Layers: Since I practice chair yoga indoors, I like to wear layers that I can easily remove if I start to feel too warm. A light, breathable top paired with leggings or loose pants works perfectly for me. If it's chilly, I can always throw on a cozy sweater or shawl to stay warm.

5. Mind the Length: I pay attention to the length of my clothing, especially my pants or leggings. I want to make sure they're not too long or too loose, as I don't want them to bunch up or get in the way during my practice. Ankle-length leggings or pants that hit just below the knee are usually my go-to choices.

6. Choose Supportive Undergarments: It's important to wear supportive undergarments that provide enough coverage and support during our practice. A comfortable sports bra and seamless underwear are my go-to choices— they keep everything in place without digging into my skin or causing any discomfort.

7. Accessorize Wisely: When it comes to accessories, I keep it minimal. I like to wear a comfortable headband to keep my hair out of my face and a simple bracelet or necklace for a touch of personal style. However, I avoid wearing anything too bulky or distracting that might get in the way during my practice.

8. Consider Footwear: Since chair yoga is done while sitting down, footwear isn't usually necessary. However, if you prefer to wear shoes for extra support or traction, opt for comfortable, non-slip shoes with a flexible sole that allows for natural movement.

9. Personal Style: Lastly, I always remember to embrace my personal style when choosing my yoga outfit. Whether it's a favorite color, pattern, or style of clothing, I like to wear something that makes me feel confident and happy— it's all about expressing myself and feeling good during my practice!

Above are some tips for picking the perfect outfit for chair yoga! With comfortable, breathable fabrics, loose-fitting clothing, and supportive undergarments, you'll be ready to rock your practice in style. Remember to listen to your body and choose clothing that makes you feel comfortable and confident— it's all about enjoying the journey and feeling good in your own skin.

Warmups And Breathing Exercises

1. Gentle Shoulder Rolls: I love starting my warm-up routine with gentle shoulder rolls. Sitting comfortably in my chair, I roll my shoulders forward in big circles, then backward. It feels amazing to release any tension and loosen up my shoulders before moving into other stretches.

2. Arm Circles: Next, I like to do some arm circles to wake up my upper body. With my arms extended out to the sides, I make small circles with my fingertips, gradually increasing the size of the circles as I go. This helps improve circulation and flexibility in my arms and shoulders.

3. Neck Stretches: To release tension in my neck and improve mobility, I do some gentle neck stretches. Sitting tall in my chair, I slowly tilt my head to one side, bringing my ear towards my shoulder until I feel a gentle stretch along the side of my neck. Then, I switch to the other side. I repeat this movement a few times, moving slowly and mindfully.

4. Deep Breathing: Now, let's move on to some breathing exercises. One of my favorites is deep belly breathing. I place one hand on my chest and the other on my belly, then take a slow, deep breath in through my nose, feeling my belly rise as I fill my lungs with air. Then, I exhale slowly through my mouth, feeling my belly fall. This helps me feel calm and centered, and it's great for reducing stress and anxiety.

5. Counted Breathing: Another breathing exercise I enjoy is counted breathing. I inhale slowly for a count of four, then hold my breath for a count of four, and exhale slowly for a count of four. It's like a mini meditation that helps me focus my mind and regulate my breathing.

6. Alternate Nostril Breathing: For a more advanced breathing exercise, I like to practice alternate nostril breathing. I use my thumb to close off one nostril, then inhale deeply through the other nostril. Then, I switch sides, closing off the other nostril with my ring finger and exhaling through the first nostril. This helps balance my energy and promote relaxation.

7. Mindful Body Scan: Finally, I like to end my warm-up and breathing routine with a mindful body scan. I close my eyes and take a few moments to tune into my body, noticing any areas of tension or discomfort. Then, I gently bring my awareness to each part of my body, starting with my toes and working my way up to the top of my head. This helps me feel grounded and present in the moment.

FOUNDATIONAL POSES AND TECHNIQUES

1. Seated Mountain Pose:

- Sit tall in your chair with your feet flat on the ground and your hands resting on your thighs.

- Take a moment to find your alignment— align your ears over your shoulders and your shoulders over your hips.

- Engage your core muscles by gently drawing your belly button towards your spine.

- Lift your chest and lengthen your spine, imagining a string pulling you up towards the ceiling.

- Relax your shoulders down away from your ears and soften your facial muscles.

- Close your eyes if it feels comfortable and take a few deep breaths, focusing on lengthening your spine with each inhale and relaxing any tension with each exhale.

- Hold the pose for 30 seconds to 1 minute, breathing deeply and mindfully.

2. Seated Cat-Cow Stretch:

- Sit tall in your chair with your feet flat on the ground and your hands resting on your thighs.

- Inhale as you arch your back, lifting your chest and tilting your pelvis forward (this is the "Cow" position).

- Exhale as you round your spine, tucking your chin towards your chest and pressing your hands into your thighs (this is the "Cat" position).

- Continue moving between Cat and Cow pose with your breath, inhaling as you arch your back and exhaling as you round your spine.

- Focus on moving smoothly and gently, feeling the stretch in your spine and the muscles along your back.

- Repeat for 5-10 rounds, moving slowly and mindfully with each breath.

3. Seated Forward Fold:

- Sit tall in your chair with your feet flat on the ground and your hands resting on your thighs.

- Inhale as you lengthen your spine and lift your chest.

- Exhale as you hinge forward at your hips, leading with your chest and reaching your hands towards your feet or the floor.

- Keep your back straight and your neck in line with your spine— avoid rounding your back or straining your neck.

- Only fold forward as far as feels comfortable, stopping when you feel a gentle stretch in the back of your legs and lower back.

- Hold the forward fold for 15-30 seconds, breathing deeply and relaxing into the stretch.

- To come out of the pose, inhale as you slowly rise back up to a seated position, stacking your vertebrae one by one.

4. Seated Side Stretch:

- Sit tall in your chair with your feet flat on the ground and your hands resting on your thighs.

- Inhale as you reach your right arm up towards the ceiling, lengthening through your fingertips.

- Exhale as you lean to the left, stretching your right arm over your head and reaching towards the left side of the room.

- Keep both hips grounded on the chair and both feet flat on the ground— avoid leaning to one side or lifting your hips.

- Feel the stretch along the right side of your body, from your fingertips down to your hip.

- Hold the stretch for 15-30 seconds, breathing deeply and feeling the expansion in your ribcage with each inhale.

- To come out of the pose, inhale as you slowly return to an upright seated position, then repeat on the other side.

5. Seated Twist:

- Sit tall in your chair with your feet flat on the ground and your hands resting on your thighs.

- Inhale as you lengthen your spine and lift your chest.

- Exhale as you twist to the right, placing your left hand on the outside of your right thigh and your right hand on the back of the chair.

- Keep both hips grounded on the chair and both feet flat on the ground— avoid lifting your hips or straining your back.

- Gently twist from your waist, using your breath to deepen the stretch with each exhale.

- Hold the twist for 15-30 seconds, breathing deeply and feeling the rotation in your spine.

- To come out of the pose, inhale as you slowly return to an upright seated position, then repeat on the other side.

6. Seated Shoulder Rolls:

- Sit comfortably in your chair with your feet flat on the ground and your hands resting on your thighs.

- Inhale as you lift your shoulders up towards your ears, scrunching them up tightly.

- Exhale as you roll your shoulders back and down in a smooth, circular motion.

- Continue rolling your shoulders in a circular motion for 5-10 rounds, then reverse the direction of the circles.

- Focus on releasing any tension or tightness in your shoulders with each roll, allowing your breath to guide the movement.

7. Seated Neck Stretches:

- Sit tall in your chair with your feet flat on the ground and your hands resting on your thighs.

- Inhale as you lengthen your spine and lift your chest.

- Exhale as you gently tilt your head to the right, bringing your right ear towards your right shoulder.

- Hold the stretch for 15-30 seconds, feeling a gentle stretch along the left side of your neck.

- Inhale as you return your head to an upright position, then exhale as you repeat the stretch on the left side.

- Continue alternating sides for 2-3 rounds, moving slowly and mindfully with each stretch.

8. Seated Spinal Twist:

- Sit tall in your chair with your feet flat on the ground and your hands resting on your thighs.

- Inhale as you lengthen your spine and lift your chest.

- Exhale as you twist to the right, placing your left hand on the outside of your right thigh and your right hand on the back of the chair.

- Use your hands to gently guide the twist, moving from your waist and keeping your spine long.

- Hold the twist for 15-30 seconds, breathing deeply and feeling the rotation in your spine.

- Inhale as you return to an upright seated position, then exhale as you repeat the twist on the left side.

- Continue alternating sides for 2-3 rounds, moving with your breath and enjoying the gentle stretch.

9. Seated Warrior I:

- Sit tall in your chair with your feet flat on the ground and your hands resting on your thighs.

- Inhale as you lengthen your spine and lift your chest.

- Exhale as you step your right foot back behind you, keeping your toes pointed forward and your heel lifted.

- Bend your left knee slightly, bringing it directly over your ankle.

- Inhale as you reach your arms overhead, bringing your palms together.

- Hold the pose for 15-30 seconds, feeling a stretch in the front of your right hip and thigh.

- Exhale as you release the pose, returning your right foot to the ground and bringing your arms back down to your sides.

- Repeat on the other side, stepping your left foot back and stretching your left hip and thigh.

10. Seated Warrior II:

- Sit tall in your chair with your feet flat on the ground and your hands resting on your thighs.

- Inhale as you lengthen your spine and lift your chest.

- Exhale as you step your right foot back behind you, keeping your toes pointed to the side and your heel lifted.

- Bend your left knee, bringing it directly over your ankle.

- Extend your arms out to the sides at shoulder height, parallel to the ground, with your palms facing down.

- Gaze over your left fingertips, feeling strong and grounded in the pose.

- Hold the pose for 15-30 seconds, breathing deeply and feeling the strength and stability in your legs and core.

- Exhale as you release the pose, returning your right foot to the ground and bringing your arms back down to your sides.

- Repeat on the other side, stepping your left foot back and stretching your left hip and thigh.

11. Seated Warrior III:

- Sit tall in your chair with your feet flat on the ground and your hands resting on your thighs.

- Inhale as you lengthen your spine and lift your chest.

- Exhale as you lean forward slightly, lifting your right leg off the ground and extending it straight back behind you.

- Keep your left foot firmly planted on the ground and engage your core to help you balance.

- Reach your arms out in front of you, parallel to the ground, with your palms facing each other.

- Keep your hips square to the front of the chair and your torso parallel to the ground.

- Hold the pose for 15-30 seconds, breathing deeply and feeling the strength and stability in your core and standing leg.

- Exhale as you release the pose, returning your right foot to the ground and bringing your arms back down to your sides.

- Repeat on the other side, lifting your left leg and extending it straight back behind you.

12. Seated Tree Pose:

- Sit tall in your chair with your feet flat on the ground and your hands resting on your thighs.

- Shift your weight into your left foot and bring the sole of your right foot to rest on your inner left thigh, just above your knee.

- Press your right foot into your left thigh and your left thigh into your right foot to create a stable base.

- Bring your hands together at your heart center in a prayer position, or extend your arms overhead with your palms facing each other.

- Engage your core muscles to help you balance and find a focal point to gaze at to help you stay steady.

- Hold the pose for 15-30 seconds, breathing deeply and feeling rooted and grounded like a tree.

- Repeat on the other side, bringing your left foot to rest on your inner right thigh.

13. Seated Eagle Arms:

- Sit tall in your chair with your feet flat on the ground and your hands resting on your thighs.

- Inhale as you extend your arms out to the sides at shoulder height, parallel to the ground.

- Exhale as you cross your right arm over your left arm, bringing your palms together in front of your face.

- If possible, hook your right elbow under your left elbow and bring the backs of your hands together.

- If this is too intense, simply press the palms of your hands together in front of your face.

- Lift your elbows slightly and draw your shoulder blades down your back, feeling a stretch across your upper back and shoulders.

- Hold the pose for 15-30 seconds, breathing deeply and feeling the opening in your chest and shoulders.

- Release the pose on an exhale, then repeat with your left arm crossing over your right arm.

14. Seated Sun Salutation Variation:

- Sit tall in your chair with your feet flat on the ground and your hands resting on your thighs.

- Inhale as you sweep your arms overhead, reaching up towards the ceiling.

- Exhale as you hinge forward at your hips, folding your torso over your thighs and reaching towards your feet or the floor.

- Inhale as you lengthen your spine and lift your chest halfway, coming into a flat back position.

- Exhale as you fold forward again, bringing your hands back to the floor or resting them on your thighs.

- Inhale as you sweep your arms out to the sides and up overhead, coming back to an upright seated position.

- Exhale as you bring your hands back down to your thighs, returning to your starting position.

- Repeat this sequence 3-5 times, moving with your breath and enjoying the gentle flow of movement.

15. Seated Child's Pose - Breathing Techniques:

- Sit tall in your chair with your feet flat on the ground and your hands resting on your thighs.

- Inhale deeply through your nose, filling your belly with air and expanding your ribcage.

- Exhale slowly and completely through your mouth, allowing your chest and belly to deflate.

- On your next inhale, reach your arms forward and hinge forward at your hips, bringing your torso towards your thighs.

- Allow your forehead to rest on the back of your hands or on a cushion placed on your thighs.

- Close your eyes and focus on your breath, feeling the rise and fall of your belly with each inhale and exhale.

- Hold the pose for 5-10 deep breaths, allowing yourself to surrender and relax into the stretch.

- To come out of the pose, slowly sit back up and return to an upright seated position, taking a moment to notice how you feel.

BUILDING STRENGTH AND FLEXIBILITY

1. Seated Leg Lifts:

- Sit tall in your chair with your feet flat on the ground and your hands resting on your thighs.

- Engage your core muscles by gently drawing your belly button towards your spine.

- Inhale as you lengthen your spine and lift your chest.

- Exhale as you extend one leg straight out in front of you, keeping your foot flexed.

- Hold the leg up for a few seconds, then inhale as you lower it back down to the ground.

- Repeat on the other side, alternating legs for a total of 8-10 repetitions on each side.

- Focus on keeping your core engaged and your back straight throughout the movement.

2. Seated Knee Lifts:

- Sit tall in your chair with your feet flat on the ground and your hands resting on your thighs.

- Inhale as you lift one knee towards your chest, bringing it as close to your body as comfortable.

- Exhale as you lower the foot back down to the ground.

- Repeat on the other side, alternating legs for a total of 8-10 repetitions on each side.

- Focus on keeping your back straight and your shoulders relaxed throughout the movement.

3. Seated Leg Extensions:

- Sit tall in your chair with your feet flat on the ground and your hands resting on your thighs.

- Inhale as you extend one leg straight out in front of you, keeping your foot flexed.

- Exhale as you lower the foot back down to the ground.

- Repeat on the other side, alternating legs for a total of 8-10 repetitions on each side.

- Focus on keeping your core engaged and your back straight throughout the movement.

4. Seated Heel Raises:

- Sit tall in your chair with your feet flat on the ground and your hands resting on your thighs.

- Inhale as you lift your heels off the ground, rising up onto the balls of your feet.

- Exhale as you lower your heels back down to the ground.

- Repeat for a total of 8-10 repetitions, moving slowly and mindfully with each lift and lower.

- Focus on keeping your ankles steady and your knees aligned over your ankles throughout the movement.

5. Seated Hip Openers:

- Sit tall in your chair with your feet flat on the ground and your hands resting on your thighs.

- Inhale as you bring one ankle up to rest on the opposite knee, creating a figure-four shape with your legs.

- Exhale as you gently press down on the raised knee, feeling a stretch in the hip of the raised leg.

- Hold the stretch for 15-30 seconds, breathing deeply and relaxing into the stretch.

- Release the stretch and repeat on the other side, alternating legs for a total of 2-3 stretches on each side.

6. Seated Chair Pose:

- Sit tall in your chair with your feet flat on the ground and your hands resting on your thighs.

- Inhale as you reach your arms overhead, bringing your biceps alongside your ears.

- Exhale as you bend your knees and lower your hips back and down as if you were sitting in an invisible chair.

- Keep your weight in your heels and your knees aligned over your ankles.

- Hold the pose for 15-30 seconds, breathing deeply and engaging your core and leg muscles.

- To come out of the pose, inhale as you slowly rise back up to a standing position, bringing your arms back down to your sides.

7. Seated Side Leg Lifts:

- Sit tall in your chair with your feet flat on the ground and your hands resting on your thighs.

- Inhale as you lift one leg straight out to the side, keeping it parallel to the ground.

- Exhale as you lower the leg back down to the ground.

- Repeat on the other side, alternating legs for a total of 8-10 repetitions on each side.

- Focus on keeping your core engaged and your back straight throughout the movement.

- You can also hold onto the sides of the chair for added stability if needed.

8. Seated Figure Four Stretch:

- Sit tall in your chair with your feet flat on the ground and your hands resting on your thighs.

- Inhale as you bring one ankle up to rest on the opposite knee, creating a figure-four shape with your legs.

- Exhale as you gently press down on the raised knee, feeling a stretch in the hip of the raised leg.

- Hold the stretch for 15-30 seconds, breathing deeply and relaxing into the stretch.

- Release the stretch and repeat on the other side, alternating legs for a total of 2-3 stretches on each side.

- Keep your back straight and avoid rounding your spine as you fold forward.

9. Seated Hamstring Stretch:

- Sit tall in your chair with your feet flat on the ground and your hands resting on your thighs.

- Extend one leg straight out in front of you, keeping your foot flexed.

- Inhale as you lengthen your spine and lift your chest.

- Exhale as you hinge forward at your hips, reaching towards your toes or the shin of your extended leg.

- Hold the stretch for 15-30 seconds, breathing deeply and feeling the stretch in the back of your extended leg.

- Keep your back straight and avoid rounding your spine as you fold forward.

- Repeat on the other side, alternating legs for a total of 2-3 stretches on each side.

10. Seated Calf Stretch:

- Sit tall in your chair with your feet flat on the ground and your hands resting on your thighs.

- Extend one leg straight out in front of you, keeping your foot flexed.

- Inhale as you lengthen your spine and lift your chest.

- Exhale as you gently pull your toes back towards your body, feeling a stretch in your calf muscle.

- Hold the stretch for 15-30 seconds, breathing deeply and relaxing into the stretch.

- Release the stretch and repeat on the other side, alternating legs for a total of 2-3 stretches on each side.

- Keep your back straight and avoid rounding your spine as you perform the stretch.

11. Seated Quadriceps Stretch:

- Sit tall in your chair with your feet flat on the ground and your hands resting on your thighs.

- Extend one leg straight out in front of you, keeping your foot flexed.

- Inhale as you lengthen your spine and lift your chest.

- Exhale as you gently bend the opposite knee and bring your heel towards your buttocks, grabbing onto your ankle or foot with your hand.

- Hold the stretch for 15-30 seconds, feeling the stretch in the front of your thigh.

- Keep your knees close together and avoid arching your lower back as you perform the stretch.

- Release the stretch and repeat on the other side, alternating legs for a total of 2-3 stretches on each side.

12. Seated Chest Opener:

- Sit tall in your chair with your feet flat on the ground and your hands resting on your thighs.

- Inhale as you interlace your fingers behind your back, squeezing your shoulder blades together.

- Exhale as you gently lift your hands away from your body, opening your chest and lifting your gaze towards the ceiling.

- Hold the stretch for 15-30 seconds, breathing deeply and feeling the expansion in your chest and shoulders.

- Keep your shoulders relaxed and avoid scrunching them up towards your ears.

- Release the stretch and repeat for 2-3 rounds, focusing on opening up your chest with each breath.

13. Seated Backbend:

- Sit tall in your chair with your feet flat on the ground and your hands resting on your thighs.

- Inhale as you sweep your arms overhead, reaching up towards the ceiling.

- Exhale as you lean back slightly, arching your spine and lifting your chest towards the sky.

- Keep your shoulders relaxed and avoid crunching your lower back— focus on opening up through your upper back and chest.

- Hold the backbend for 15-30 seconds, breathing deeply and feeling the stretch in your spine.

- To come out of the pose, inhale as you slowly return to an upright seated position, bringing your arms back down to your sides.

14. Seated Side Bend:

- Sit tall in your chair with your feet flat on the ground and your hands resting on your thighs.

- Inhale as you reach your right arm up overhead, lengthening through your fingertips.

- Exhale as you gently lean to the left, stretching the right side of your body.

- Keep both hips grounded on the chair and both feet flat on the ground— avoid lifting your hips or leaning too far to one side.

- Hold the stretch for 15-30 seconds, breathing deeply and feeling the lengthening sensation along the right side of your body.

- Inhale as you return to an upright seated position, then repeat on the other side, reaching your left arm up and leaning to the right.

15. Seated Forward Bend:

- Sit tall in your chair with your feet flat on the ground and your hands resting on your thighs.

- Inhale as you lengthen your spine and lift your chest.

- Exhale as you hinge forward at your hips, leading with your chest and reaching your hands towards your feet or the floor.

- Keep your back straight and your neck in line with your spine— avoid rounding your back or straining your neck.

- Only fold forward as far as feels comfortable, stopping when you feel a gentle stretch in the back of your legs and lower back.

- Hold the forward bend for 15-30 seconds, breathing deeply and relaxing into the stretch.

- To come out of the pose, inhale as you slowly rise back up to a seated position, stacking your vertebrae one by one.

BALANCING AND ALIGNMENT

1. Seated Mountain Pose with Arms Extended:

- Sit tall in your chair with your feet flat on the ground and your hands resting on your thighs.

- Inhale as you sweep your arms overhead, reaching up towards the ceiling.

- Exhale as you extend your arms out to the sides, bringing your biceps alongside your ears.

- Engage your core muscles by gently drawing your belly button towards your spine.

- Hold the pose for 15-30 seconds, breathing deeply and feeling the stretch in your arms and sides.

- Keep your shoulders relaxed and your spine lengthened throughout the pose.

2. Seated Knee Squeezes with Core Engagement:

- Sit tall in your chair with your feet flat on the ground and your hands resting on your thighs.

- Inhale deeply as you engage your core muscles by pulling your belly button towards your spine.

- Exhale as you gently squeeze your knees together, engaging the muscles of your inner thighs.

- Hold the squeeze for a few seconds, feeling the activation in your core.

- Release the squeeze on an inhale, then repeat for a total of 8-10 repetitions.

- Focus on maintaining good posture and breathing deeply throughout the exercise.

3. Seated Leg Cross with Twist:

- Sit tall in your chair with your feet flat on the ground and your hands resting on your thighs.

- Cross your right leg over your left thigh, placing your right foot on the ground next to your left knee.

- Inhale as you lengthen your spine and lift your chest.

- Exhale as you twist to the right, placing your left hand on your right knee and your right hand on the back of the chair.

- Hold the twist for 15-30 seconds, breathing deeply and feeling the stretch in your spine.

- Inhale as you slowly return to an upright seated position, then repeat on the other side.

4. Seated Side Stretch with Arm Reach:

- Sit tall in your chair with your feet flat on the ground and your hands resting on your thighs.

- Inhale as you reach your right arm up overhead, lengthening through your fingertips.

- Exhale as you gently lean to the left, stretching the right side of your body.

- Hold the stretch for 15-30 seconds, breathing deeply and feeling the lengthening sensation along the right side of your body.

- Inhale as you return to an upright seated position, then repeat on the other side, reaching your left arm up and leaning to the right.

5. Seated Tree Pose with Hand on Heart:

- Sit tall in your chair with your feet flat on the ground and your hands resting on your thighs.

- Place your right foot on the inside of your left thigh, just above your knee, or keep it on the ground for a modified version.

- Bring your hands together at your heart center, or place your right hand on your heart and your left hand on top of your right hand.

- Close your eyes if it feels comfortable and take a few deep breaths, feeling the connection between your hand and your heart.

- Hold the pose for 15-30 seconds, breathing deeply and feeling grounded and centered.

6. Seated Eagle Arms with Twist:

- Sit tall in your chair with your feet flat on the ground and your hands resting on your thighs.

- Inhale as you extend your arms out to the sides at shoulder height, parallel to the ground.

- Exhale as you cross your right arm over your left arm, bringing your palms together in front of your face.

- If possible, hook your right elbow under your left elbow and bring the backs of your hands together.

- Inhale deeply and lengthen through your spine.

- Exhale as you twist to the left, bringing your elbows towards your left knee.

- Hold the twist for 15-30 seconds, breathing deeply and feeling the stretch in your upper back and shoulders.

- Inhale as you slowly release the twist and return to an upright seated position, then repeat on the other side.

7. Seated Figure Four Stretch with Forward Fold:

- Sit tall in your chair with your feet flat on the ground and your hands resting on your thighs.

- Cross your right ankle over your left thigh, creating a figure-four shape with your legs.

- Flex your right foot to protect your knee.

- Inhale deeply as you lengthen your spine and lift your chest.

- Exhale as you hinge forward at your hips, leading with your chest and reaching towards your feet or the floor.

- Keep your back straight and your neck in line with your spine— avoid rounding your back or straining your neck.

- Hold the forward fold for 15-30 seconds, breathing deeply and relaxing into the stretch.

- Inhale as you slowly rise back up to an upright seated position, then repeat on the other side.

8. Seated Warrior II with Gaze Focus:

- Sit tall in your chair with your feet flat on the ground and your hands resting on your thighs.

- Extend your right leg out to the side, keeping your foot flat on the ground.

- Rotate your torso to the right, bringing your right arm forward and your left arm back.

- Gaze over your right fingertips, keeping your neck long and your chin parallel to the ground.

- Engage your core muscles and press firmly into the ground with your feet for stability.

- Hold the pose for 15-30 seconds, breathing deeply and feeling strong and grounded.

- Repeat on the other side, extending your left leg out to the side and rotating your torso to the left.

9. Seated Half Moon Pose with Side Stretch:

- Sit tall in your chair with your feet flat on the ground and your hands resting on your thighs.

- Extend your right arm overhead, reaching up towards the ceiling.

- Inhale deeply as you lengthen through your fingertips.

- Exhale as you gently lean to the left, stretching the right side of your body.

- Keep your hips grounded on the chair and your feet flat on the ground.

- Hold the stretch for 15-30 seconds, breathing deeply and feeling the lengthening sensation along the right side of your body.

- Inhale as you return to an upright seated position, then repeat on the other side, reaching your left arm up and leaning to the right.

10. Seated Boat Pose with Leg Lifts:

- Sit tall in your chair with your feet flat on the ground and your hands resting on your thighs.

- Inhale deeply as you engage your core muscles and lift both legs off the ground, bringing your knees towards your chest.

- Exhale as you extend your legs out in front of you, keeping them lifted and parallel to the ground.

- Keep your spine long and your chest lifted, and avoid rounding your back.

- Hold the pose for 15-30 seconds, breathing deeply and feeling the engagement in your core and legs.

- If it feels comfortable, you can extend your arms forward alongside your legs.

- Release the pose on an exhale and lower your feet back to the ground.

11. Seated Twist with Arm Bind:

- Sit tall in your chair with your feet flat on the ground and your hands resting on your thighs.

- Inhale deeply as you lengthen your spine and lift your chest.

- Exhale as you twist to the right, bringing your left hand to the outside of your right knee and your right hand behind your back.

- If possible, reach your right hand around your back and clasp your left hand, binding your arms together.

- Keep your spine long and your shoulders relaxed, and avoid rounding your back.

- Hold the twist for 15-30 seconds, breathing deeply and feeling the rotation in your spine.

- Inhale as you slowly release the twist and return to an upright seated position, then repeat on the other side.

12. Seated Dancer Pose with Arm Extension:

- Sit tall in your chair with your feet flat on the ground and your hands resting on your thighs.

- Extend your right arm overhead, reaching up towards the ceiling.

- Bend your left knee and reach back with your left hand to grab onto the outside of your left foot or ankle.

- Inhale deeply as you lengthen through your right fingertips and lift your chest.

- Exhale as you gently press your foot into your hand, opening up through the front of your body.

- Hold the pose for 15-30 seconds, breathing deeply and feeling the stretch in your chest and shoulders.

- Release the pose on an exhale and repeat on the other side, extending your left arm overhead and grabbing onto your right foot or ankle with your right hand.

13. Seated Forward Fold with Shoulder Opener:

- Sit tall in your chair with your feet flat on the ground and your hands resting on your thighs.

- Inhale deeply as you lengthen your spine and lift your chest.

- Exhale as you hinge forward at your hips, leading with your chest and reaching towards your feet or the floor.

- Keep your back straight and your neck in line with your spine— avoid rounding your back or straining your neck.

- If it feels comfortable, reach your arms behind your back and interlace your fingers, opening up through your shoulders.

- Hold the forward fold for 15-30 seconds, breathing deeply and relaxing into the stretch.

- Inhale as you slowly rise back up to an upright seated position.

14. Seated Side Plank with Hip Lift:

- Sit tall in your chair with your feet flat on the ground and your hands resting on your thighs.

- Place your right hand on the seat of the chair next to your right hip, fingers pointing towards your feet.

- Inhale deeply as you engage your core muscles and lift your hips off the chair, coming into a side plank position.

- Keep your body in a straight line from your head to your heels, and avoid letting your hips sink or lift too high.

- Hold the pose for 15-30 seconds, breathing deeply and feeling the engagement in your core and side body.

- Exhale as you lower your hips back down to the chair, then repeat on the other side, placing your left hand on the chair and lifting your hips.

15. Seated Warrior III with Leg Extension:

- Sit tall in your chair with your feet flat on the ground and your hands resting on your thighs.

- Extend your right leg straight out in front of you, keeping your foot flexed.

- Inhale deeply as you lengthen your spine and lift your chest.

- Exhale as you hinge forward at your hips, reaching your arms out in front of you and lifting your left leg off the ground.

- Keep your hips squared towards the front of the chair and your torso parallel to the ground.

- Hold the pose for 15-30 seconds, breathing deeply and feeling the engagement in your core and standing leg.

- Inhale as you slowly return to an upright seated position, then repeat on the other side, extending your left leg and lifting your right leg.

CHAIR YOGA FOR SPECIFIC CONDITIONS

Chair yoga can be tailored to address specific health conditions, making it accessible and beneficial for people with various needs.

1. Arthritis: Chair yoga offers gentle movements that can help alleviate stiffness and pain associated with arthritis. Poses are modified to reduce strain on joints while improving flexibility and range of motion. Gentle stretches and breathing exercises can also help manage arthritis symptoms by promoting relaxation and reducing stress.

2. Osteoporosis: For individuals with osteoporosis, chair yoga focuses on gentle weight-bearing exercises to help maintain bone density and prevent fractures. Poses are modified to avoid forward bends and twisting motions that could strain the spine. Strengthening exercises for the legs, hips, and core help improve balance and stability, reducing the risk of falls.

3. Chronic Pain: Chair yoga provides a safe and accessible way to manage chronic pain conditions such as fibromyalgia or lower back pain. Gentle stretches and mindful movements can help alleviate tension in muscles and promote relaxation. Breathing techniques and meditation practices incorporated into chair yoga sessions can also help reduce stress and improve overall well-being.

4. Heart Disease: Chair yoga can be beneficial for individuals with heart disease by promoting gentle cardiovascular exercise and stress reduction. Modified yoga poses help improve circulation and lower blood pressure, reducing the risk of heart-related complications. Breathing exercises and relaxation techniques can also help manage anxiety and promote heart health.

5. Multiple Sclerosis (MS): Chair yoga offers a supportive and adaptable practice for individuals with MS, focusing on gentle movements and mindfulness. Poses are modified to accommodate fatigue, weakness, and balance issues commonly associated with MS. Chair yoga helps improve mobility, coordination, and overall quality of life for individuals living with MS.

6. Anxiety and Depression: Chair yoga provides a therapeutic outlet for managing symptoms of anxiety and depression. Mindful movement, deep breathing exercises, and relaxation techniques help reduce stress levels and promote a sense of calmness and emotional well-being. Chair yoga classes offer a supportive community environment where individuals can connect and share their experiences.

Overall, chair yoga is a versatile and inclusive practice that can be adapted to meet the needs of individuals with specific health conditions. Whether it's arthritis, osteoporosis, chronic pain, heart disease, MS, anxiety, or depression, chair yoga offers gentle movements, breathwork, and relaxation techniques to support physical, emotional, and mental well-being.

Arthritis Exercises:

1. Seated Neck Rolls:

  - Sit comfortably in a chair with your feet flat on the ground and your hands resting on your thighs.

  - Inhale as you gently drop your right ear towards your right shoulder, feeling a stretch along the left side of your neck.

  - Exhale as you roll your chin towards your chest, feeling a stretch along the back of your neck.

- Inhale as you roll your left ear towards your left shoulder, feeling a stretch along the right side of your neck.

- Continue this gentle rolling motion for 5-10 repetitions, moving with your breath and taking care not to strain your neck.

2. Seated Shoulder Rolls:

- Sit comfortably in a chair with your feet flat on the ground and your hands resting on your thighs.

- Inhale as you lift your shoulders up towards your ears, squeezing them tightly.

- Exhale as you roll your shoulders back and down, opening up your chest and squeezing your shoulder blades together.

- Continue this rolling motion for 5-10 repetitions, moving with your breath and focusing on releasing tension in your shoulders.

3. Seated Cat-Cow Stretch:

- Sit comfortably in a chair with your feet flat on the ground and your hands resting on your thighs.

- Inhale as you arch your back and lift your chest towards the ceiling, coming into a gentle backbend (Cow Pose).

- Exhale as you round your spine and tuck your chin towards your chest, dropping your head down towards your chest (Cat Pose).

4. Seated Forward Fold:

- Sit comfortably in a chair with your feet flat on the ground and your hands resting on your thighs.

- Inhale as you lengthen your spine and lift your chest.

- Exhale as you hinge forward at your hips, reaching your hands towards your feet or the floor.

- Allow your head to hang heavy and relax your neck and shoulders.

- Hold the forward fold for 15-30 seconds, breathing deeply and feeling the stretch along the back of your legs and spine.

5. Seated Twist:

- Sit comfortably in a chair with your feet flat on the ground and your hands resting on your thighs.

- Inhale as you lengthen your spine and lift your chest.

- Exhale as you twist to the right, placing your left hand on your right knee and your right hand on the back of the chair.

- Use your breath to deepen the twist with each exhale, gently rotating your spine.

- Hold the twist for 15-30 seconds, breathing deeply and feeling the stretch along your spine and sides.

- Inhale as you return to center, then repeat on the other side, twisting to the left.

6. Seated Ankle Circles:

- Sit comfortably in a chair with your feet flat on the ground.

- Inhale as you lift your right foot off the ground, flexing your right ankle.

- Exhale as you circle your right foot clockwise, making slow and controlled movements.

- After several circles, reverse the direction and circle your right foot counterclockwise.

- Repeat the ankle circles for 5-10 repetitions, then switch to your left foot and repeat the sequence.

Osteoporosis Exercisess:

1. Seated Shoulder Rolls:

- Sit comfortably in a chair with your feet flat on the ground and your hands resting on your thighs.

- Inhale deeply as you lift your shoulders up towards your ears, tensing the muscles in your shoulders.

- Exhale as you roll your shoulders back and down in a circular motion, opening up your chest.

- Continue rolling your shoulders in a circular motion for 5-10 repetitions, then reverse the direction.

2. Seated Cat-Cow Stretch:

- Sit comfortably in a chair with your feet flat on the ground and your hands resting on your thighs.

- Inhale deeply as you arch your back and lift your chest towards the ceiling, allowing your belly to drop towards your thighs (Cow Pose).

- Exhale as you round your back, tucking your chin towards your chest and drawing your belly button towards your spine (Cat Pose).

- Continue flowing between Cow Pose and Cat Pose with your breath for 5-10 repetitions, focusing on the movement of your spine.

3. Seated Forward Fold with Bent Knees:

- Sit comfortably in a chair with your feet flat on the ground and your hands resting on your thighs.

- Inhale deeply as you lengthen your spine and lift your chest.

- Exhale as you hinge forward at your hips, keeping a slight bend in your knees to protect your spine.

- Reach your hands towards your feet or the floor, allowing your head to hang heavy and relaxing your neck and shoulders.

- Hold the forward fold for 15-30 seconds, breathing deeply and feeling the stretch along the back of your legs and spine.

4. Seated Side Stretch with Gentle Arm Reach:

- Sit comfortably in a chair with your feet flat on the ground and your hands resting on your thighs.

- Inhale deeply as you reach your right arm overhead, lengthening through your fingertips.

- Exhale as you gently lean to the left, feeling a stretch along the right side of your body.

- Hold the stretch for a few breaths, then inhale as you return to center and repeat on the other side.

5. Seated Spinal Twist with Support:

- Sit comfortably in a chair with your feet flat on the ground and your hands resting on your thighs.

- Inhale deeply and lengthen your spine, sitting tall.

- Exhale as you twist gently to the right, placing your left hand on the outside of your right knee and your right hand on the back of the chair for support.

- Hold the twist for a few breaths, feeling the stretch along the sides of your body.

- Inhale as you return to center, then repeat the twist on the other side, twisting to the left.

6. Seated Neck Stretches with Gentle Head Tilts:

- Sit comfortably in a chair with your feet flat on the ground and your hands resting on your thighs.

- Inhale deeply and lengthen your spine, sitting tall.

- Exhale as you gently tilt your head to the right, bringing your right ear towards your right shoulder.

- Hold the stretch for a few breaths, feeling the stretch along the left side of your neck.

- Inhale as you return to center, then repeat the stretch on the other side, tilting your head to the left.

Heart Disease Exercises:

1. Seated Neck Stretches:

- Sit comfortably in a chair with your feet flat on the ground and your hands resting on your thighs.

- Inhale deeply and lengthen your spine, sitting tall.

- Exhale as you gently tilt your head to the right, bringing your right ear towards your right shoulder.

- Hold the stretch for a few breaths, feeling the stretch along the left side of your neck.

- Inhale as you return to center, then repeat the stretch on the other side, tilting your head to the left.

2. Seated Shoulder Rolls:

- Sit comfortably in a chair with your feet flat on the ground and your hands resting on your thighs.

- Inhale deeply as you lift your shoulders up towards your ears, tensing the muscles in your shoulders.

- Exhale as you roll your shoulders back and down in a circular motion, opening up your chest.

- Continue rolling your shoulders in a circular motion for 5-10 repetitions, then reverse the direction.

3. Seated Side Stretch:

- Sit comfortably in a chair with your feet flat on the ground and your hands resting on your thighs.

- Inhale deeply as you raise your right arm overhead, reaching up towards the ceiling.

- Exhale as you gently lean to the left, feeling a stretch along the right side of your body.

- Hold the stretch for a few breaths, then inhale as you return to center and repeat on the other side.

4. Seated Cat-Cow Stretch:

- Sit comfortably in a chair with your feet flat on the ground and your hands resting on your thighs.

- Inhale deeply as you arch your back and lift your chest towards the ceiling, allowing your belly to drop towards your thighs (Cow Pose).

- Exhale as you round your back, tucking your chin towards your chest and drawing your belly button towards your spine (Cat Pose).

- Continue flowing between Cow Pose and Cat Pose with your breath for 5-10 repetitions, focusing on the movement of your spine.

5. Seated Forward Fold:

- Sit comfortably in a chair with your feet flat on the ground and your hands resting on your thighs.

- Inhale deeply as you lengthen your spine and lift your chest.

- Exhale as you hinge forward at your hips, reaching your hands towards your feet or the floor.

- Allow your head to hang heavy and relax your neck and shoulders.

- Hold the forward fold for 15-30 seconds, breathing deeply and feeling the stretch along the back of your legs and spine.

6. Seated Breathing Exercises:

- Sit comfortably in a chair with your feet flat on the ground and your hands resting on your thighs.

- Close your eyes and take a few deep breaths, inhaling through your nose and exhaling through your mouth.

- As you breathe, focus on expanding your chest and filling your lungs with air.

- Practice deep breathing for 2-3 minutes, feeling your body relax with each breath.

RELAXATION AND STRESS RELIEF

Relaxation and stress relief are essential for maintaining overall well-being. It involves techniques and practices aimed at reducing tension in both the body and mind. Relaxation techniques can include deep breathing exercises, progressive muscle relaxation, guided imagery, and mindfulness meditation. By engaging in these practices, individuals can lower their heart rate, decrease muscle tension, and promote a sense of calmness and tranquility.

Stress relief techniques help individuals manage and alleviate the negative effects of stress on the body and mind. These techniques may involve physical activities such as yoga, tai chi, or gentle exercise, which can help release endorphins and improve mood. Additionally, engaging in hobbies, spending time in nature, and connecting with loved ones are effective ways to reduce stress levels. By incorporating relaxation and stress relief techniques into daily routines, individuals can improve their overall quality of life and better cope with the challenges of everyday stressors.

Relaxation Techniques

1. Deep Breathing:

  - Sit or lie down comfortably in a quiet space.

  - Close your eyes and take a slow, deep breath in through your nose, counting to four.

  - Hold your breath for a moment, then exhale slowly through your mouth, counting to six.

  - As you exhale, imagine releasing any tension or stress from your body.

- Repeat this deep breathing pattern for several minutes, focusing on each inhale and exhale.

2. Progressive Muscle Relaxation:

- Start by tensing the muscles in your forehead and scalp by squeezing them tightly for a few seconds.

- Then, slowly release the tension and notice the sensation of relaxation spreading through your forehead and scalp.

- Continue this process, moving down to your eyes, jaw, neck, shoulders, arms, hands, chest, abdomen, back, hips, legs, and feet, tensing and relaxing each muscle group one at a time.

3. Guided Imagery:

- Find a comfortable position and close your eyes.

- Imagine yourself in a peaceful place, such as a beach, forest, or mountain.

- Picture the scene in detail, focusing on sensory experiences like the sound of waves, the smell of pine trees, or the feeling of soft sand beneath your feet.

- Spend a few minutes immersing yourself in this imaginary environment, allowing yourself to feel calm and relaxed.

4. Mindfulness Meditation:

- Sit or lie down comfortably and bring your attention to your breath.

- Notice the sensation of each inhale and exhale, focusing on the rise and fall of your chest or the feeling of air passing through your nostrils.

- When thoughts or distractions arise, gently acknowledge them without judgment and return your focus to your breath.

- Practice this mindful awareness for a few minutes, gradually increasing the duration as you become more comfortable with the practice.

5. Yoga and Tai Chi:

- Follow along with a beginner-friendly yoga or Tai Chi video or class.

- Pay attention to your breath as you move through gentle stretches and poses, focusing on each movement and the sensations in your body.

- Allow yourself to relax into each pose, using deep breathing to deepen the stretch and release tension.

- Enjoy the flow of movement and the sense of peace and calm that comes with practicing these ancient mind-body exercises.

6. Aromatherapy:

- Choose a calming essential oil, such as lavender, chamomile, or eucalyptus.

- Place a few drops of the oil into a diffuser or onto a cotton ball and inhale deeply.

- Alternatively, add a few drops of the oil to a warm bath or massage oil for a soothing sensory experience.

- Allow the calming aroma to fill the room and help you relax and unwind.

Progressive Muscle Relaxation (PMR)

Progressive Muscle Relaxation (PMR) is a relaxation technique that involves systematically tensing and then relaxing different muscle groups in the body to reduce physical tension and induce a state of relaxation. Here's how to practice PMR in simple steps:

1. Find a Comfortable Position: Sit or lie down in a comfortable and quiet space where you won't be disturbed. Close your eyes if it helps you to relax.

2. Begin with Breathing: Take a few slow, deep breaths to help calm your mind and prepare for the practice.

3. Start with Tension: Begin by tensing one muscle group at a time. Start with your forehead and scrunch up your forehead muscles tightly for about 5-10 seconds. Focus on the sensation of tension in your forehead.

4. Release Tension: After tensing the muscle group, slowly and gently release the tension while exhaling. Pay attention to the feeling of relaxation spreading through the muscle. Let go of any remaining tension as you relax.

5. Move Through Muscle Groups: Continue this process, moving systematically through different muscle groups in your body. Progress through the following sequence, holding each tension for 5-10 seconds before releasing:

   - Forehead

- Jaw

- Neck and shoulders

- Arms and hands

- Chest and abdomen

- Back

- Hips and buttocks

- Thighs

- Calves

- Feet

6. Focus on Sensations: As you tense and release each muscle group, pay attention to the sensations of tension and relaxation. Notice how it feels when the muscle is tense versus when it's relaxed.

7. Practice Regularly: Repeat the process of tensing and relaxing each muscle group 2-3 times, or as desired. Practice PMR regularly, ideally once or twice a day, to experience its full benefits.

8. End with Deep Breathing: After completing the sequence, take a few deep breaths and allow yourself to fully relax. Take a moment to notice how your body feels now compared to before you started.

<u>**Stress Management**</u>

1. Deep Breathing:

   - Step 1: Find a quiet and comfortable place to sit or lie down.

   - Step 2: Close your eyes and take a slow, deep breath in through your nose, counting to four.

   - Step 3: Hold your breath for a moment, then exhale slowly through your mouth, counting to six.

   - Step 4: Repeat this deep breathing pattern for a few minutes, focusing on each inhale and exhale to calm your mind and body.

2. Mindfulness Meditation:

   - Step 1: Sit or lie down comfortably and close your eyes.

   - Step 2: Bring your attention to your breath, noticing the sensation of each inhale and exhale.

   - Step 3: When thoughts or distractions arise, gently acknowledge them without judgment and return your focus to your breath.

   - Step 4: Practice this mindful awareness for a few minutes, gradually increasing the duration as you become more comfortable with the practice.

3. Exercise:

   - Step 1: Choose an activity you enjoy, such as walking, jogging, or dancing.

- Step 2: Set aside time each day to engage in physical exercise, even if it's just for a short duration.

- Step 3: Focus on moving your body and releasing built-up tension and stress through movement.

- Step 4: Notice how exercise makes you feel afterward, and aim to incorporate it into your routine regularly for maximum benefits.

4. Healthy Lifestyle Choices:

- Step 1: Prioritize getting enough sleep each night, aiming for 7-9 hours of quality sleep.

- Step 2: Eat a balanced diet rich in fruits, vegetables, whole grains, and lean proteins to fuel your body and support overall well-being.

- Step 3: Limit caffeine, alcohol, and processed foods, which can contribute to stress and anxiety.

- Step 4: Take breaks throughout the day to rest and recharge, engaging in activities you enjoy and spending time with loved ones.

5. Time Management:

- Step 1: Make a list of tasks and prioritize them based on importance and urgency.

- Step 2: Break larger tasks into smaller, more manageable steps to prevent feeling overwhelmed.

- Step 3: Use tools like calendars, planners, or apps to schedule your time effectively and avoid procrastination.

- Step 4: Remember to schedule time for relaxation and self-care activities to maintain balance in your life.

Guided Journaling

Certainly! Guided journaling is a therapeutic practice that involves using prompts or questions to guide your writing and exploration of thoughts, feelings, and experiences. Here's how to practice guided journaling in simple steps:

1. Choose a Journal: Select a notebook or journal that you feel comfortable using. It can be plain or decorative, lined or blank, depending on your preference.

2. Set Aside Time: Find a quiet and comfortable space where you won't be interrupted. Set aside dedicated time for journaling, whether it's in the morning, evening, or during a break in your day.

3. Select a Prompt: Choose a prompt or question to focus your journaling session. Prompts can vary widely and may relate to self-reflection, gratitude, goal-setting, or emotional processing.

4. Reflect and Write: Begin writing in response to the prompt, allowing your thoughts and feelings to flow freely onto the page. Write without judgment or censoring yourself, and don't worry about grammar or spelling.

5. Explore Emotions: Use the journaling process to explore and process your emotions. Notice any patterns or recurring themes in your writing, and reflect on how you're feeling in the present moment.

6. Express Gratitude: Consider incorporating gratitude journaling into your practice by writing about things you're thankful for each day. This can help shift your focus toward positivity and appreciation.

7. Set Intentions: Use guided journaling as an opportunity to set intentions or goals for yourself. Write about what you want to accomplish and how you plan to achieve it, breaking down your goals into actionable steps.

8. Review and Reflect: Periodically review your journal entries to track your progress, gain insights into your thoughts and behaviors, and celebrate your achievements. Reflect on how journaling has impacted your well-being and growth.

9. Experiment and Adapt: Explore different prompts, writing styles, and journaling techniques to find what resonates best with you. Don't be afraid to experiment and adapt your practice based on your changing needs and interests.

10. Enjoy the Process: Remember that guided journaling is a personal and creative practice meant to support your well-being and self-discovery. Enjoy the process of writing and exploring your inner world, and be gentle with yourself along the way.

SPECIAL CONSIDERATIONS

Modifications For Seniors

1. Low-Impact Exercises: Instead of high-impact activities like running or jumping, I focus on low-impact exercises that are gentler on my joints. This can include activities like walking, swimming, or cycling, which provide cardiovascular benefits without putting too much strain on my body.

2. Chair-Based Exercises: Sometimes standing exercises can be challenging, so I incorporate chair-based exercises into my routine. These exercises allow me to work on strength, flexibility, and balance while seated in a sturdy chair. For example, I might do seated leg lifts, arm curls with light weights, or seated twists to engage my core.

3. Balance and Stability Training: As we age, maintaining balance and stability becomes increasingly important to prevent falls and injuries. I incorporate exercises that focus on balance and stability, such as standing on one leg, heel-to-toe walking, or using balance boards or stability balls. These exercises help improve proprioception and reduce the risk of falls.

4. Flexibility Exercises: Keeping my muscles and joints flexible is essential for maintaining mobility and preventing stiffness. I include regular stretching exercises in my routine to improve flexibility and range of motion. This can include stretches for the neck, shoulders, back, hips, and legs, holding each stretch for 15-30 seconds without bouncing.

5. Gradual Progression: I've learned the importance of starting slowly and gradually increasing the intensity or duration of my workouts. This allows my body to adapt and prevents overexertion or injury. I listen to my body and pay attention to any signs of fatigue or discomfort, adjusting my workout accordingly.

6. Proper Form and Alignment: I focus on maintaining proper form and alignment during exercises to prevent strain or injury. This means paying attention to my posture, engaging the right muscles, and moving in a controlled manner. I also make sure to warm up before exercising and cool down afterwards to prepare my body and prevent stiffness.

7. Listen to My Body: Above all, I listen to my body and respect its limits. If something doesn't feel right or if I experience pain or discomfort, I take a break or modify the exercise as needed. I've learned to tune into my body's signals and adjust my workouts accordingly to ensure a safe and enjoyable experience.

By incorporating these modifications into my exercise routine, I'm able to stay active, healthy, and independent as a senior. It's important to remember that exercise should be enjoyable and sustainable, so finding activities that I love and that suit my needs is key to maintaining a lifelong fitness routine.

Chair Support Options

When it comes to sitting comfortably, having the right support is essential. There are various chair support options available to ensure that you can sit comfortably and safely. Let me break them down for you:

1. Back Support: Back support is crucial for maintaining good posture and preventing discomfort or pain in the lower back. Many chairs come with built-in lumbar support, which helps support the natural curve of the spine. If your chair doesn't have built-in lumbar support, you can use a lumbar pillow or cushion to provide additional support to your lower back.

2. Seat Cushions: Seat cushions can help provide extra padding and support for your bottom and thighs, making sitting for extended periods more comfortable. Gel seat cushions, memory foam cushions, or even simple foam cushions can help distribute your weight more evenly and reduce pressure on your hips and tailbone.

3. Armrests: Armrests are designed to provide support for your arms and shoulders while sitting. They can help reduce strain on your shoulders and neck by providing a place to rest your arms. Adjustable armrests are ideal because they allow you to customize the height and width of the armrests to fit your body comfortably.

4. Footrests: Footrests are particularly important if your feet don't comfortably reach the ground when sitting. They can help improve circulation and reduce pressure on your legs by providing support for your feet and legs. Adjustable footrests are ideal because they allow you to adjust the height and angle to find the most comfortable position for your legs.

5. Headrests: Headrests are designed to support your head and neck while sitting, reducing strain on your neck and shoulders. They can be particularly beneficial if you spend long hours sitting at a desk or computer. Look for chairs with adjustable headrests that allow you to customize the height and angle for optimal support.

6. Posture Correctors: Posture correctors are devices that attach to your chair and help promote proper posture while sitting. They typically work by encouraging you to sit upright and align your spine correctly. Some posture correctors may include adjustable straps or cushions to provide additional support where needed.

7. Ergonomic Chairs: Ergonomic chairs are designed to support the natural curves of your spine and promote good posture while sitting. They often come with adjustable features such as seat height, backrest angle, and armrest height to accommodate different body types and preferences. Investing in an ergonomic chair can provide long-term comfort and support, especially if you spend a lot of time sitting.

Having the right chair support options can make a significant difference in your comfort and well-being while sitting. Whether you're working at a desk, relaxing at home, or dining at the table, choosing chairs with adequate support can help prevent discomfort and promote better posture. Experiment with different support options to find what works best for you, and don't hesitate to invest in quality chairs that prioritize your comfort and health.

Seated vs. Standing Variations

When it comes to yoga or exercise routines, you might have noticed that some poses or movements can be done either while sitting down or standing up. Each variation has its own benefits and considerations, and choosing between them depends on factors like comfort, mobility, and personal preference.

Seated poses are done while sitting on a chair or on the floor with your legs crossed or extended in front of you. These variations are great for people who may have difficulty standing for long periods, have limited mobility, or prefer a gentler approach to exercise.

One of the benefits of seated variations is that they provide support and stability, making them ideal for beginners or those with balance issues. Since you're already seated, there's less risk of losing your balance or straining your muscles, which can be reassuring, especially if you're new to yoga or exercise.

Seated variations also allow for greater accessibility. You can easily practice yoga or do exercises from a seated position, whether you're at home, in the office, or anywhere else with a chair. This makes it convenient to incorporate movement into your daily routine without needing a lot of space or equipment.

Another advantage of seated variations is that they can help reduce strain on the joints and lower back. By sitting down, you're taking pressure off your knees, hips, and spine, which can be beneficial if you have joint pain or stiffness. Seated poses also provide an opportunity to focus on stretching and strengthening specific muscle groups without putting undue stress on other parts of the body.

On the other hand, standing variations offer a different set of benefits. Standing poses are done while standing upright on both feet, with or without the support of a chair or other props. These variations are great for improving balance, building strength, and increasing flexibility.

One of the main advantages of standing variations is that they engage more muscles and require greater stability. When you're standing, you're using your legs, core, and even your arms to support your body weight and maintain proper alignment. This can help improve overall strength and coordination over time.

Standing variations also encourage better posture and spinal alignment. By standing tall and engaging your core muscles, you can help alleviate back pain and improve your overall posture, which is important for preventing injuries and maintaining mobility as you age.

Additionally, standing variations offer a greater range of motion and challenge compared to seated poses. Since you're working against gravity, standing exercises can help improve balance and proprioception, which is your body's awareness of its position in space. This can be especially beneficial for older adults or anyone looking to improve their balance and stability.

Both seated and standing variations have their own unique benefits and considerations. Seated poses offer support, accessibility, and joint relief, while standing poses promote strength, balance, and posture. Depending on your needs and preferences, you can choose to incorporate a combination of seated and standing variations into your yoga or exercise routine for a well-rounded and effective workout.

INCORPORATING YOGA INTO DAILY LIFE

1. Start the Day with Yoga:

Every morning, I carve out a few minutes to practice yoga. It doesn't have to be long - even just 10-15 minutes of gentle stretching and breathing exercises can set a positive tone for the day ahead. I focus on poses that awaken my body and calm my mind, such as Child's Pose, Cat-Cow Stretch, and Sun Salutations.

2. Take Yoga Breaks:

Throughout the day, I take short breaks to do quick yoga poses or stretches. Whether I'm sitting at my desk or standing in line at the grocery store, I find moments to reconnect with my breath and release tension from my body. Simple stretches like Neck Rolls, Shoulder Shrugs, and Seated Twists help me stay centered and focused amidst the busyness of life.

3. Practice Mindful Movement:

As I go about my daily activities, I try to move mindfully and with intention. Whether I'm walking, cooking, or doing household chores, I pay attention to my body and how it feels in each moment. I use the principles of yoga - like awareness of breath and alignment - to move with grace and ease, preventing strain and injury.

4. Embrace Yoga Off the Mat:

Yoga isn't just about physical poses - it's a way of living that extends beyond the mat. I strive to embody the values of yoga in my interactions with others and in how I approach challenges. I practice compassion, patience, and gratitude in my daily life, knowing that these qualities are essential for inner peace and well-being.

5. Find Moments of Stillness:

In the midst of a busy day, I make time for moments of stillness and reflection. Whether it's sitting quietly with a cup of tea or taking a few deep breaths outside, I cherish these moments of peace and solitude. They allow me to recharge and reconnect with myself, fostering a sense of inner calm and clarity.

6. End the Day with Relaxation:

Before bed, I wind down with gentle yoga poses and relaxation techniques. I focus on releasing any tension or stress from my body, preparing myself for a restful night's sleep. Poses like Legs-Up-the-Wall, Supine Twist, and Savasana help me let go of the day's worries and surrender to a state of deep relaxation.

By integrating yoga into my daily life in these ways, I cultivate greater mindfulness, balance, and well-being. Yoga becomes not just something I do, but a way of being - guiding me towards greater peace, vitality, and harmony in all aspects of my life.

INTEGRATING MINDFULNESS INTO DAILY ACTIVITIES

Integrating mindfulness into daily activities is a powerful way to bring more awareness and presence into our lives. It's about being fully engaged and attentive to the present moment, no matter what we're doing. Here's how I integrate mindfulness into my daily activities:

1. Morning Routine: As I wake up in the morning, I take a moment to focus on my breath. I pay attention to the sensation of air entering and leaving my body, grounding myself in the present moment before I start my day. As I brush my teeth or take a shower, I bring my awareness to the sensations and movements involved, savoring the simple acts of self-care.

2. Eating Mindfully: During meals, I try to eat slowly and pay attention to the flavors, textures, and smells of my food. I chew each bite mindfully, savoring the experience and appreciating the nourishment it provides. By eating without distractions, such as TV or phone, I can fully enjoy my meals and listen to my body's hunger and fullness cues.

3. Walking Mindfully: Whether I'm walking to work or taking a stroll in nature, I practice walking mindfully. I focus on the sensation of my feet touching the ground, the movement of my muscles, and the sights and sounds around me. I let go of any distractions or racing thoughts and simply enjoy the act of walking.

4. Mindful Work: In my work or daily tasks, I strive to be fully present and engaged. I break tasks down into smaller steps and focus on one thing at a time,

giving it my full attention. I take short breaks to pause, breathe, and check in with myself, allowing me to recharge and approach my work with clarity and intention.

5. Mindful Communication: When interacting with others, I practice mindful communication. I listen attentively, without interrupting or judging, and respond thoughtfully rather than reactively. I pay attention to my body language and tone of voice, striving to communicate with kindness, empathy, and authenticity.

6. Mindful Relaxation: In moments of relaxation, such as reading a book or listening to music, I allow myself to fully immerse in the experience. I let go of any worries or distractions and focus on the present moment, finding joy and peace in simple pleasures.

7. Mindful Evening Routine: As the day comes to a close, I wind down with a mindful evening routine. I take time to reflect on my day, acknowledging both the challenges and moments of gratitude. I practice relaxation techniques, such as deep breathing or gentle stretching, to prepare my body and mind for restful sleep.

By integrating mindfulness into my daily activities, I cultivate a greater sense of awareness, presence, and peace in my life. It helps me navigate life's ups and downs with resilience and compassion, fostering a deeper connection to myself and the world around me.

CONCLUSION

In conclusion, chair yoga offers seniors a gentle and accessible way to improve their physical and mental well-being. Through the practice of seated poses, breathing exercises, and mindfulness techniques, seniors can experience increased flexibility, strength, and relaxation without the need for strenuous movements or equipment. Chair yoga promotes overall health and vitality, while also providing a sense of community and connection for participants. By incorporating the principles of safety, accessibility, and enjoyment, this book aims to empower seniors to embrace the benefits of chair yoga and live healthier, more fulfilling lives. Whether practiced individually at home or in a group setting, chair yoga offers a pathway to greater mobility, comfort, and joy in everyday life.

SOMATIC EXERCISES FOR WEIGHT LOSS

Easy 10 minutes low impact workout to reclaim independence and loss body fat the healthy way

WHAT IS SOMATIC EXERCISES?

Somatic exercises are like a special kind of workout for your body and mind. They're all about helping you become more aware of how your body moves and feels. Imagine you're learning to dance, but instead of just following steps, you're paying close attention to every little movement you make.

When you do somatic exercises, you're not just going through the motions. You're taking the time to really feel what's happening in your body. It's like you're having a conversation with yourself, but instead of using words, you're using movements.

These exercises can be super gentle or a bit more intense, depending on what you need. Sometimes they involve stretching and bending, while other times they might focus on relaxing and releasing tension. The goal is always to help your body move better and feel better.

One cool thing about somatic exercises is that they're not just about the physical stuff. They also help you connect with your emotions and thoughts. You might notice that certain movements bring up feelings or memories. That's totally normal and actually a really important part of the process.

So why do people do somatic exercises? Well, there are lots of reasons! For starters, they can help reduce stress and anxiety. When you're really tuned in to your body, it's easier to notice when you're feeling tense or overwhelmed. Doing somatic exercises can help you relax and calm down.

These exercises can also improve your flexibility and range of motion. If you've ever felt stiff or achy, somatic exercises might be just what you need to loosen up those tight muscles and joints.

Another cool thing about somatic exercises is that they can help improve your posture and balance. When you're paying attention to how you're moving, you start to notice when things are out of whack. Over time, this can help you stand taller and feel more stable on your feet.

But maybe the best thing about somatic exercises is that they're all about listening to your body. Instead of pushing yourself to do more, faster, harder, you're learning to tune in and respond to what your body needs in the moment. It's like giving yourself permission to slow down and take care of yourself.

And here's the really awesome part: anyone can do somatic exercises! You don't need any fancy equipment or special training. All you need is a little bit of time and a willingness to pay attention to yourself.

So, whether you're looking to reduce stress, improve flexibility, or just feel more at home in your own body, somatic exercises might be worth giving a try. Who knows? You might discover a whole new way of moving and being that feels just right for you.

BENEFITS OF SOMATIC EXERCISES FOR WEIGHT LOSS

Somatic exercises are like a secret weapon for weight loss because they do more than just make you sweat. They're not about crazy cardio or heavy lifting; instead, they're all about tuning into your body and moving with intention. Here's why they're so awesome for shedding those extra pounds:

1. Increased Body Awareness: Somatic exercises help you become best friends with your body. You learn to listen to its whispers and shouts, understanding where you hold tension, stiffness, or pain. By becoming aware of these areas, you can target them with specific movements, releasing tension and promoting better movement patterns.

2. Mind-Body Connection: Imagine your body and mind holding hands and skipping through a field of daisies— that's the mind-body connection. Somatic exercises strengthen this bond, helping you understand how your thoughts and emotions affect your physical sensations. When you're more in tune with yourself, you're better equipped to make healthy choices and stick to your weight loss journey.

3. Stress Reduction: Stress and weight gain are like two peas in a pod, but somatic exercises kick stress to the curb. With deep breathing, gentle movements, and mindfulness, you can wave goodbye to tension and hello to relaxation. Lower stress levels mean lower levels of cortisol, the pesky hormone that tells your body to store fat, especially around your belly.

4. Improved Posture and Alignment: Picture yourself standing tall like a majestic oak tree— that's what good posture feels like. Somatic exercises help straighten you out by releasing tight muscles and aligning your spine. When you stand tall, you not only look slimmer but also engage your core and muscles more efficiently, burning extra calories throughout the day.

5. Better Mobility and Flexibility: You know those stiff joints that creak like an old door? Somatic exercises oil them up and get them moving smoothly again. By gently stretching and mobilizing your muscles and joints, you improve your range of motion and flexibility. Suddenly, bending down to tie your shoes or reaching for that top shelf becomes a breeze.

6. Core Strength and Stability: Your core is like the powerhouse of your body— it's where all the magic happens. Somatic exercises target your core muscles, including your abs, obliques, and lower back, making them stronger and more stable. A strong core not only supports your spine and improves posture but also helps you perform everyday activities with ease.

7. Muscle Tone and Definition: Who needs a gym full of fancy equipment when you've got your own body weight? Somatic exercises tone and sculpt your muscles, giving you that lean and defined look without the need for heavy lifting. Plus, the more muscle you have, the more calories you burn, even when you're chilling on the couch watching Netflix.

8. Boosted Metabolism: Ah, metabolism— the holy grail of weight loss. Somatic exercises rev up your metabolic engine, helping you burn more calories both during

and after your workout. As you move and groove, your body becomes a calorie-burning machine, torching fat and turning it into energy.

9. Enhanced Energy Levels: Remember that feeling of dragging yourself out of bed in the morning? Say goodbye to those days. Somatic exercises give you a natural energy boost by increasing blood flow, oxygenating your cells, and releasing feel-good endorphins. You'll feel more alive and vibrant, ready to tackle whatever the day throws your way.

10. Long-Term Weight Management: Crash diets and quick fixes? Ain't nobody got time for that. Somatic exercises teach you that slow and steady wins the race. By incorporating them into your daily routine, you build healthy habits that last a lifetime. It's not just about losing weight— it's about maintaining a balanced lifestyle that nourishes your body, mind, and soul.

SOMATIC EXERCISES

1. Cat-Cow Stretch:

- Start on your hands and knees, with your wrists directly under your shoulders and your knees under your hips.

- Inhale as you arch your back gently, lifting your head and tailbone towards the ceiling (this is the cow position).

- Exhale as you round your spine, tucking your chin to your chest and tucking your tailbone under (this is the cat position).

- Repeat these movements slowly, flowing between cat and cow positions, for about 5-10 breaths.

2. Pelvic Tilts:

- Lie on your back with your knees bent and your feet flat on the floor.

- Inhale to prepare, then exhale as you gently press your lower back into the floor by tilting your pelvis upward.

- Hold for a few seconds, then inhale as you release back to a neutral position.

- Repeat this movement, tilting your pelvis back and forth, for about 8-10 repetitions.

3. Standing Spinal Twist:

- Stand with your feet hip-width apart and your arms relaxed by your sides.

- Inhale to lengthen your spine, then exhale as you gently twist your torso to the right, placing your left hand on your right knee and your right hand on your hip or reaching behind you for support.

- Hold the twist for a few breaths, feeling the gentle stretch along your spine.

- Inhale as you return to center, then exhale and twist to the left side.

- Repeat the twist on each side 2-3 times.

4. Forward Fold:

- Stand with your feet hip-width apart and your knees slightly bent.

- Inhale to lengthen your spine, then exhale as you hinge forward at your hips, keeping your back flat.

- Allow your arms to hang towards the floor, reaching for your shins, ankles, or the floor, depending on your flexibility.

- Hold the forward fold for a few breaths, feeling the stretch in your hamstrings and lower back.

- Inhale as you slowly roll back up to standing, one vertebra at a time.

5. Seated Forward Bend:

- Sit on the floor with your legs extended straight in front of you.

- Inhale to lengthen your spine, then exhale as you hinge forward at your hips, reaching your hands towards your feet or shins.

- Keep your back straight and avoid rounding your spine excessively.

- Hold the stretch for a few breaths, feeling the gentle stretch along the back of your legs.

- Inhale as you slowly sit back up to a tall, upright position.

6. Child's Pose:

- Kneel on the floor with your big toes touching and your knees slightly apart.

- Sit back on your heels and extend your arms forward, lowering your chest towards the floor.

- Rest your forehead on the ground (or on a cushion or block if more comfortable).

- Relax your arms alongside your body or extend them forward for a deeper stretch.

- Hold the pose for 30 seconds to 1 minute, focusing on deep breathing and relaxation.

7. Shoulder Rolls:

- Sit or stand comfortably with your arms relaxed by your sides.

- Inhale as you shrug your shoulders up towards your ears.

- Exhale as you roll your shoulders back and down in a smooth, circular motion.

- Continue rolling your shoulders for 8-10 repetitions, then reverse the direction of the circles for another 8-10 repetitions.

8. Neck Stretches:

- Sit or stand comfortably with your spine tall and your shoulders relaxed.

- Inhale as you gently tilt your head to the right, bringing your right ear towards your right shoulder.

- Hold the stretch for a few breaths, feeling the gentle stretch along the left side of your neck.

- Exhale as you return to center, then repeat the stretch on the left side.

- Continue alternating between right and left neck stretches for 2-3 repetitions on each side.

9. Arm Circles:

- Stand with your feet hip-width apart and your arms extended straight out to the sides at shoulder height.

- Inhale as you circle your arms forward in a smooth, controlled motion.

- Make small circles at first, gradually increasing the size of the circles as you warm up.

- After 8-10 forward circles, reverse the direction and circle your arms backward for another 8-10 repetitions.

10. Leg Swings:

- Stand next to a sturdy support, such as a chair or wall, for balance.

- Hold onto the support with one hand for stability.

- Swing your outside leg forward and backward in a smooth, controlled motion, keeping your torso upright and your standing leg slightly bent.

- Start with small swings and gradually increase the range of motion as you feel more comfortable.

- After 8-10 swings, switch to the other leg and repeat the exercise on the opposite side.

11. Hip Circles:

- Stand with your feet hip-width apart and your hands resting on your hips.

- Slowly rotate your hips in a circular motion, starting with small circles and gradually increasing the size.

- Complete 8-10 circles in one direction, then reverse and repeat in the opposite direction.

12. Side Stretch:

- Stand tall with your feet hip-width apart and your arms relaxed by your sides.

- Reach your right arm overhead, leaning gently towards the left side to feel a stretch along the right side of your body.

- Hold the stretch for 15-30 seconds, then return to center and repeat on the other side.

13. Butterfly Stretch:

- Sit on the floor with the soles of your feet together and your knees bent out to the sides.

- Hold onto your ankles or feet with your hands.

- Gently press your knees towards the floor using your elbows while keeping your back straight.

- Hold the stretch for 15-30 seconds, feeling a gentle opening in your inner thighs.

14. Seated Twist:

- Sit on the floor with your legs extended in front of you.

- Bend your right knee and place your right foot on the outside of your left knee.

- Twist your torso to the right, placing your left elbow on the outside of your right knee and your right hand on the floor behind you for support.

- Hold the twist for 15-30 seconds, then switch sides and repeat on the other side.

15. Bridge Pose:

- Lie on your back with your knees bent and your feet hip-width apart, flat on the floor.

- Press into your feet and lift your hips towards the ceiling, engaging your glutes and core.

- Keep your shoulders relaxed and your neck long, avoiding any strain.

- Hold the pose for 15-30 seconds, then lower your hips back down to the floor.

16. Leg Raises:

- Lie on your back with your legs extended straight and your arms resting by your sides.

- Engage your core muscles and lift one leg towards the ceiling, keeping it straight.

- Lower the leg back down towards the floor without touching it, then repeat with the other leg.

- Continue alternating legs for 8-10 repetitions on each side.

17. Squats:

- Stand with your feet hip-width apart and your arms extended in front of you for balance.

- Lower your body by bending your knees and pushing your hips back as if sitting into a chair.

- Keep your chest lifted and your weight in your heels as you lower down.

- Lower as far as comfortable, then push through your heels to return to standing.

- Perform 8-10 squats, focusing on proper form and controlled movement.

18. Lunges:

- Stand with your feet hip-width apart and your hands on your hips.

- Step your right foot forward and lower your body until both knees are bent at a 90-degree angle, with your front knee aligned over your ankle.

- Keep your back straight and your chest lifted as you lunge.

- Push through your front heel to return to standing, then repeat on the other side.

- Perform 8-10 lunges on each leg, alternating sides.

19. Plank:

- Start in a push-up position with your hands directly under your shoulders and your body forming a straight line from head to heels.

- Engage your core muscles and hold this position, keeping your back flat and your hips level.

- Hold the plank for 15-30 seconds, or as long as comfortable, focusing on maintaining proper form.

- To modify, you can perform the plank on your forearms instead of your hands.

20. Side Plank:

- Start in a plank position, then shift your weight onto your right hand and outer edge of your right foot, stacking your left foot on top of your right.

- Lift your left arm towards the ceiling, creating a straight line from head to heels.

- Engage your core muscles and hold this position, keeping your hips lifted and your body in a straight line.

- Hold the side plank for 15-30 seconds, then switch sides and repeat on the other side.

Certainly! Here are step-by-step instructions for performing each exercise:

21. Boat Pose:

- Sit on the floor with your knees bent and your feet flat on the ground.

- Lean back slightly, keeping your spine straight and your chest lifted.

- Lift your feet off the ground, balancing on your sitting bones, and extend your legs out in front of you at a 45-degree angle.

- Extend your arms straight out in front of you, parallel to the ground, or hold onto the backs of your thighs for support.

- Engage your core muscles to maintain balance and hold the pose for 15-30 seconds, or as long as comfortable.

22. Mountain Climbers:

- Start in a high plank position with your hands directly under your shoulders and your body forming a straight line from head to heels.

- Engage your core muscles and drive one knee towards your chest, then quickly switch legs, alternating legs in a running motion.

- Keep your hips low and your shoulders stable as you continue to alternate legs for 30-60 seconds, or as long as comfortable.

23. Burpees:

- Begin standing with your feet hip-width apart and your arms by your sides.

- Lower into a squat position, placing your hands on the floor in front of you.

- Jump your feet back to a high plank position, keeping your body in a straight line.

- Perform a push-up by bending your elbows and lowering your chest towards the ground.

- Push through your palms to return to the plank position, then jump your feet forward towards your hands.

- Explode upwards into a jump, reaching your arms overhead.

- Land softly and immediately lower back into the squat position to begin the next repetition.

- Perform 8-10 repetitions, or as many as comfortable while maintaining good form.

24. Jumping Jacks:

- Stand with your feet together and your arms by your sides.

- Jump your feet out to the sides while simultaneously raising your arms overhead.

- Jump back to the starting position, bringing your feet together and lowering your arms by your sides.

- Continue to perform jumping jacks in a fluid motion for 30-60 seconds, or as long as comfortable.

25. High Knees:

- Stand with your feet hip-width apart and your arms bent at a 90-degree angle by your sides.

- Lift one knee towards your chest as high as possible while simultaneously raising the opposite arm.

- Quickly switch legs, alternating knees in a running motion while pumping your arms.

- Continue to alternate legs at a fast pace, bringing each knee towards your chest as high as possible, for 30-60 seconds, or as long as comfortable.

THANK YOU

Dear Valued Buyers,

As we reflect on the journey we've shared together, we're overwhelmed with gratitude for your unwavering support and trust in our products/services. Your decision to choose us among the myriad of options available speaks volumes, and we are deeply honored to have earned your business.

Your patronage not only sustains our endeavor but also fuels our passion to continually innovate and improve. Every purchase you make is a vote of confidence, motivating us to uphold the highest standards of quality, reliability, and customer satisfaction.

Beyond the transactional aspect, we cherish the connections we've forged with each of you. Your feedback, suggestions, and interactions have enriched our understanding and inspired us to strive for excellence in all that we do. It's a privilege to serve such discerning and remarkable individuals like yourselves.

As we move forward, we pledge to remain dedicated to your needs and aspirations, always seeking ways to exceed your expectations and create memorable experiences. Your continued support is the cornerstone of our success, and we are deeply grateful for the opportunity to be of service to you.

Your loyalty and trust are invaluable to us, and we look forward to many more opportunities to serve you in the future.